Awesome, Disgusting Science

GROSS SCIENCE OF DISEASES

Stephanie Bearce

Black Rabbit Books

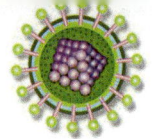
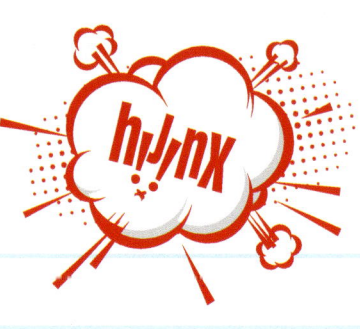

Hi Jinx is published by Black Rabbit Books
P.O. Box 227, Mankato, Minnesota, 56002.
www.blackrabbitbooks.com
Copyright © 2026 Black Rabbit Books

Alissa Thielges, editor; Jason Knudson, designer and photo researcher

All rights reserved. No part of this book may be reproduced in any form without written permission from the publisher.

Library of Congress Cataloging-in-Publication Data
Names: Bearce, Stephanie author
Title: Gross science of diseases / by Stephanie Bearce.
Description: Mankato, MN: Hi Jinx, an imprint of Black Rabbit Books, [2026] | Series: Awesome, disgusting science | Includes bibliographical references and index. | Audience: Ages 8-12 | Audience: Grades 4-6
Identifiers: LCCN 2025017495 (print) | LCCN 2025017496 (ebook) | ISBN 9781645824916 library binding | ISBN 9781645824978 paperback | ISBN 9781645825036 ebook
Subjects: LCSH: Diseases—Juvenile literature | Diseases—Research—Juvenile literature | LCGFT: Literature.
Classification: LCC R130.5 .B385 2026 (print) | LCC R130.5 (ebook) | DDC 616—dc23/eng/20250701
LC record available at https://lccn.loc.gov/2025017495

Printed in the United States of America.

Image Credits

Dreamstime/Kts, 18–19; Freepik/AI Image Creator, cover, 1, 9, 17, brgfx, 10, 11, 15, 18, 19, 23, freepik, cover, 1, 4–5, 8–9, macrovector, 8–9, 16–17, 21, storyset, cover, 1; Shutterstock/BLACKDAY, 4, Business stock, 14–15, CI Photos, 8, David Pereiras, 10–11, Dmitriy Prayzel, 18–19, Fahroni, 12, Georgy Dzyura, 7, Haninah Salsabila, 10, Kateryna Kon, 3, 13, Kwangmoozaa, 15, Memo Angeles, 20, metamorworks, 4, NikomMaelao Production, 12, nobeastsofierce, 12–13, phugunfire, 7, SB Arts Media, 4, Sinhyu Photographer, 9, SIRITAT TECHAPHALOKUL, 3, 13, Skocko, 16, 17, StockSmartStart, 6, TaraPatta, 14, thinkhubstudio, 12, 3dMediSphere, 7; Wikimedia Commons/ Piotr Smuszkiewicz, Iwona Trojanowska and Hanna Tomczak, CC BY 2.0, 16.

Every effort has been made to contact copyright holders for material reproduced in this book. Any omissions will be rectified in subsequent printings if notice is given to the publisher.

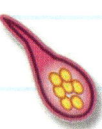
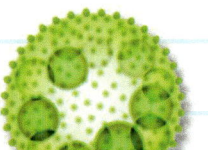

CONTENTS

CHAPTER 1
Risky Research........5

CHAPTER 2
The Experiments......6

CHAPTER 3
Get in on the Hi Jinx..20

Other Resources...........22

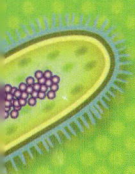
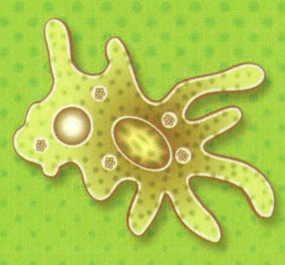
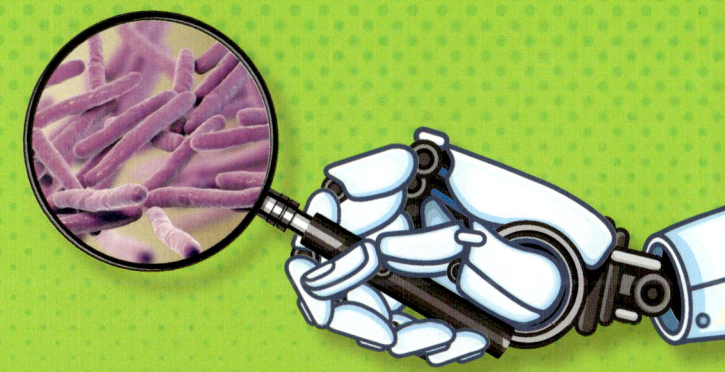
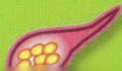

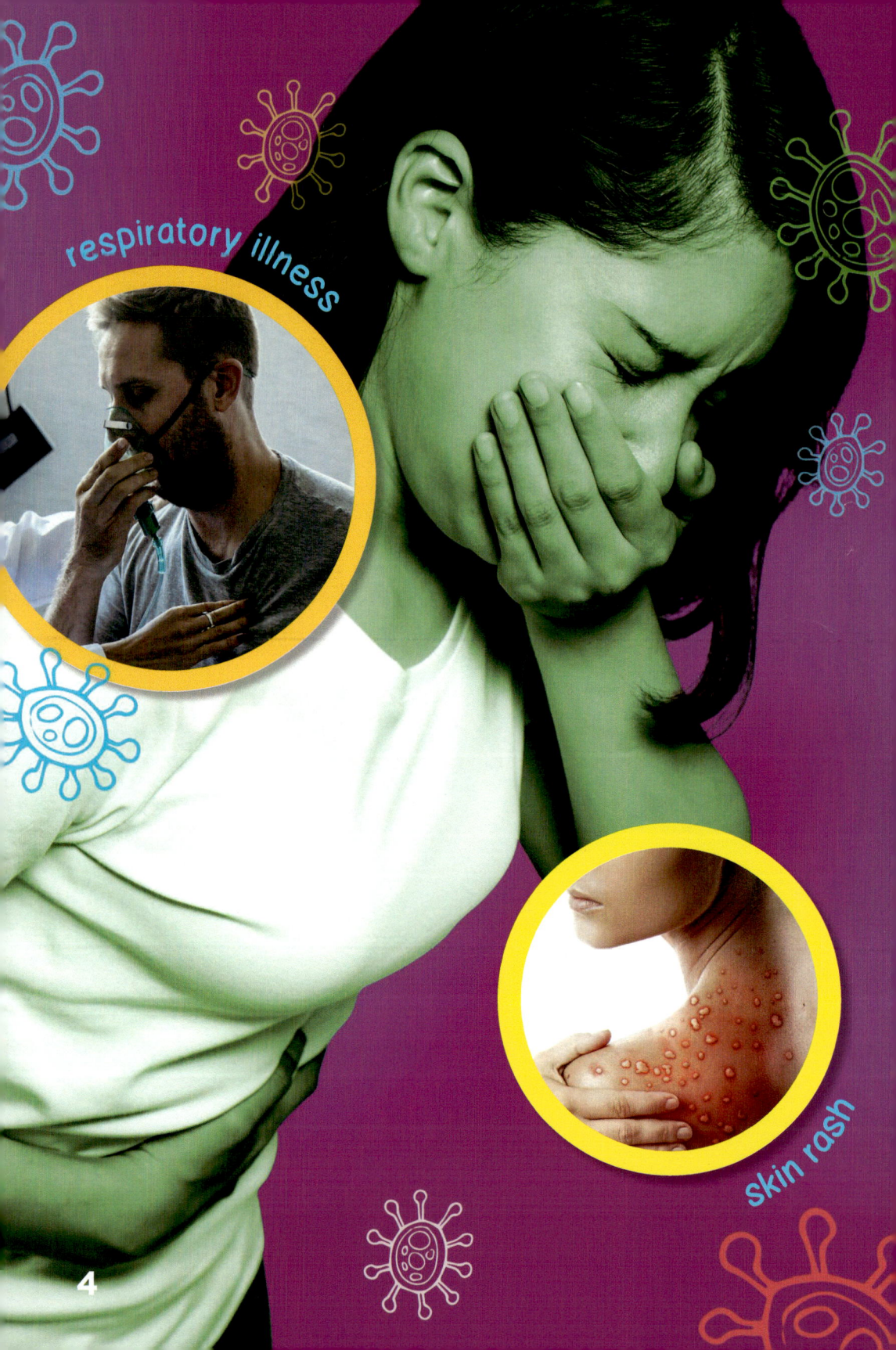

respiratory illness

skin rash

4

Chapter 1
RISKY RESEARCH

Puke and puss. Sneezes and snot. Boils and blisters. Oh gross! These are **symptoms** of diseases. Diseases come from tiny germs. They invade your body. Scientists are always searching for new ways to fight sickness. But beware! This research may come with risks.

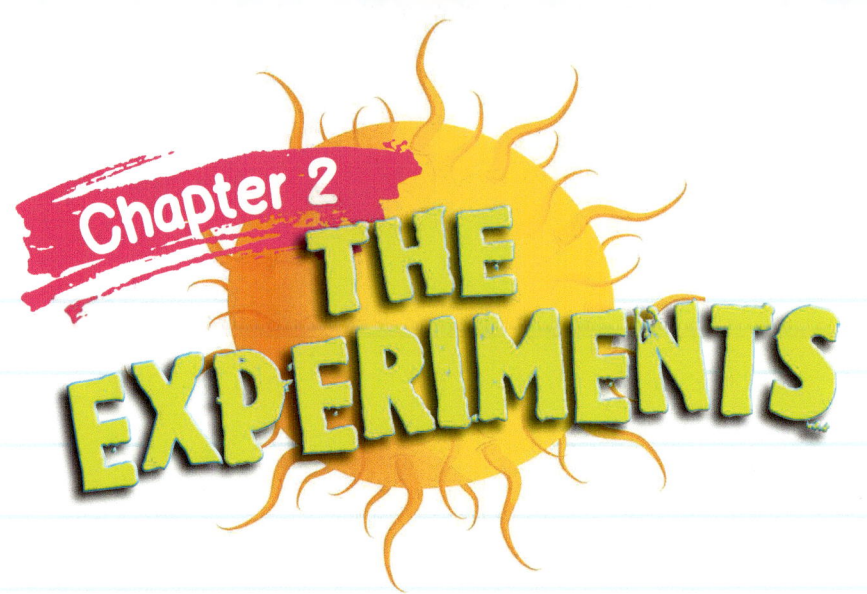

Chapter 2: THE EXPERIMENTS

Bed Buddies

Would you crawl in bed with bugs? Researchers did! Scabies are tiny mites. They cause an itchy skin disease. In one study, people with scabies slept in beds. Then people without scabies slept in the same beds. Did they get **infected**? A few did. But most did not.

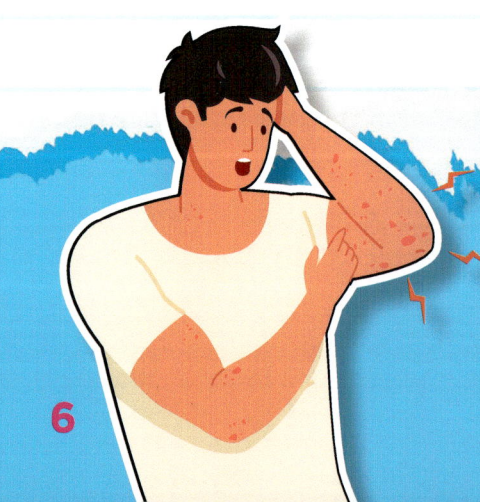

Scabies usually spread through skin contact. A special cream can zap them away.

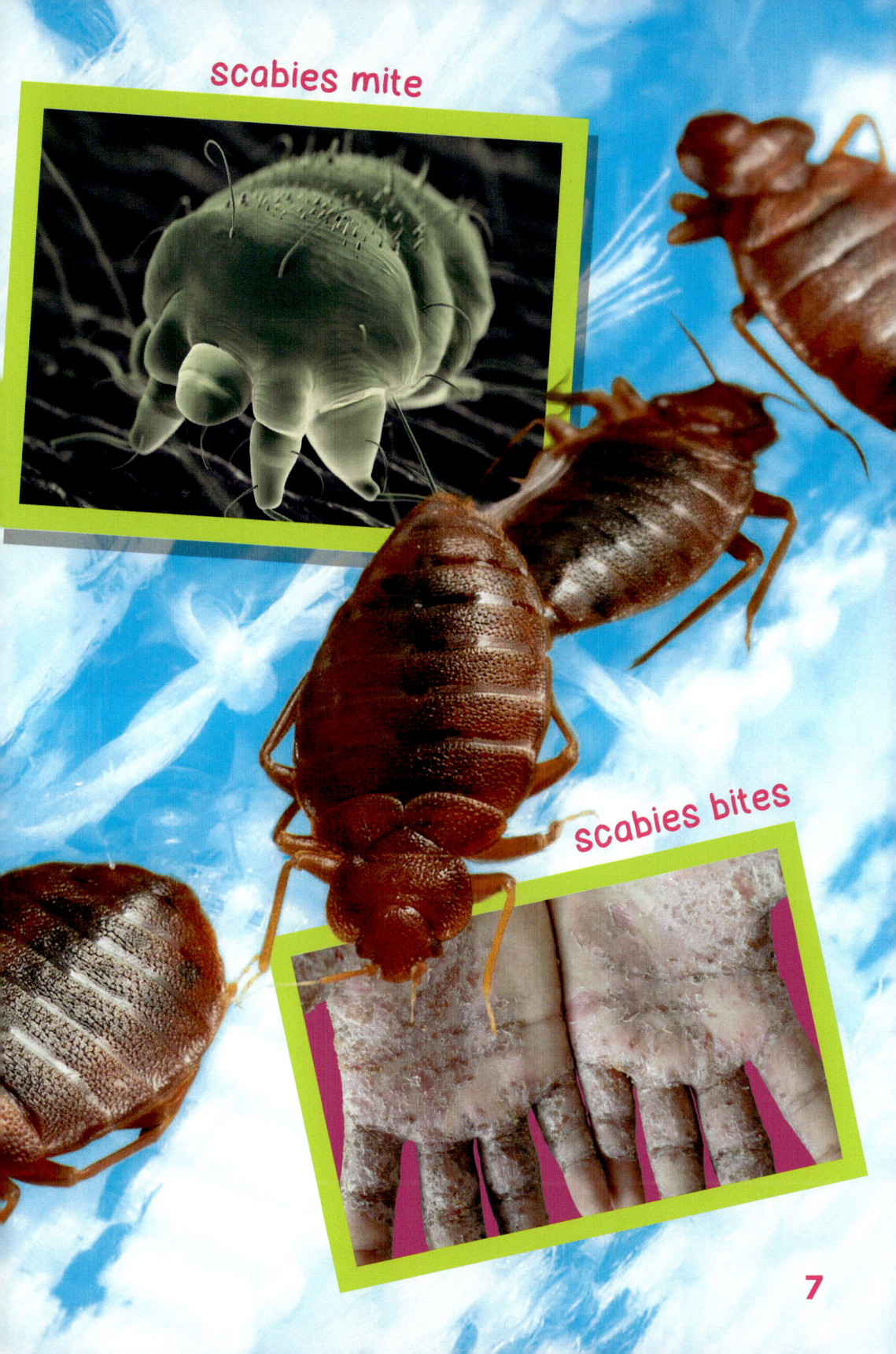

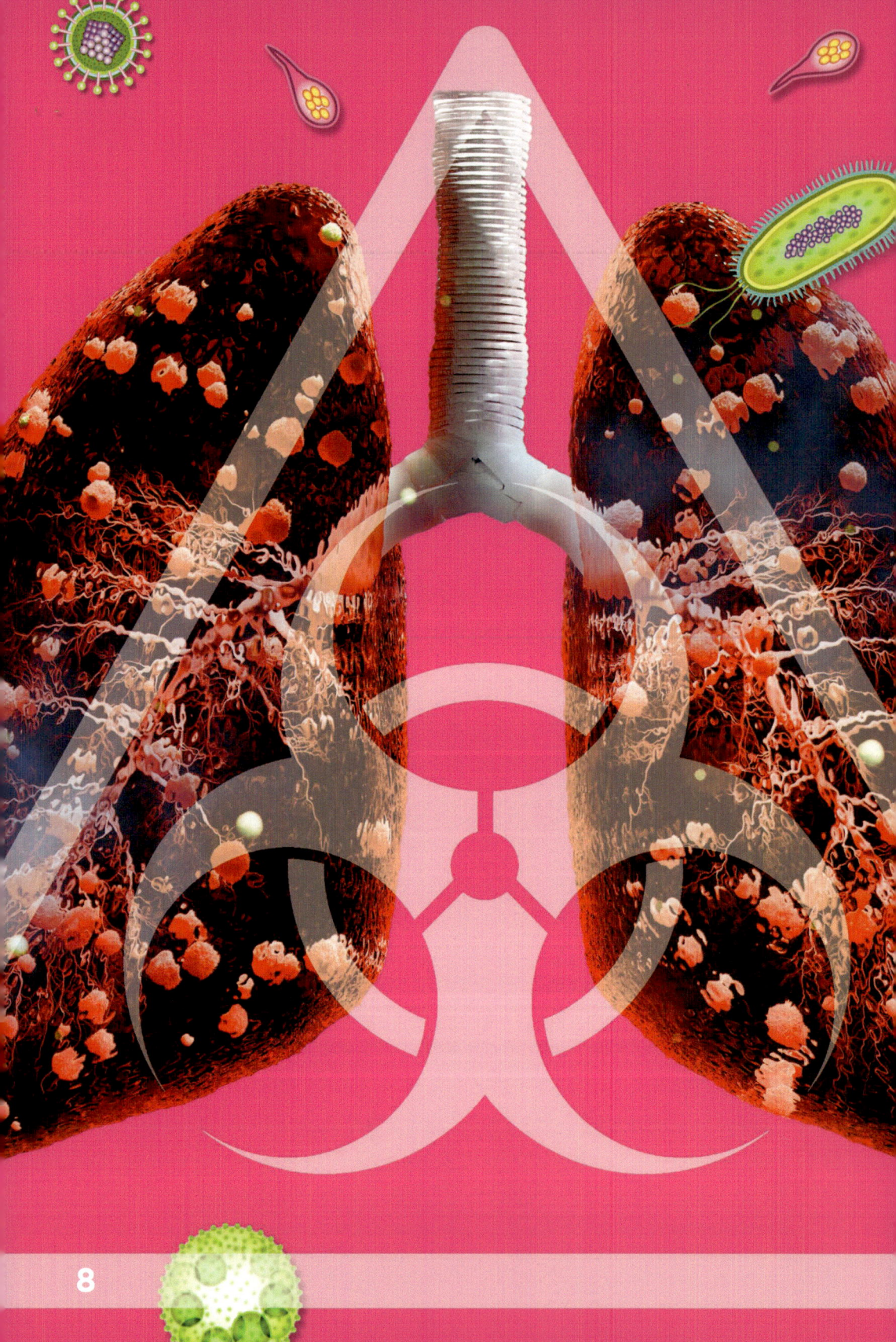

Pain Be Gone

Anthrax is bad news. Breathe it in, and it can kill you fast. It attacks your lungs and shuts down your body. But scientists found something weird. They injected mice with a tiny bit. The mice didn't feel pain! The anthrax blocked their pain signals. Could it be a new painkiller? Maybe.

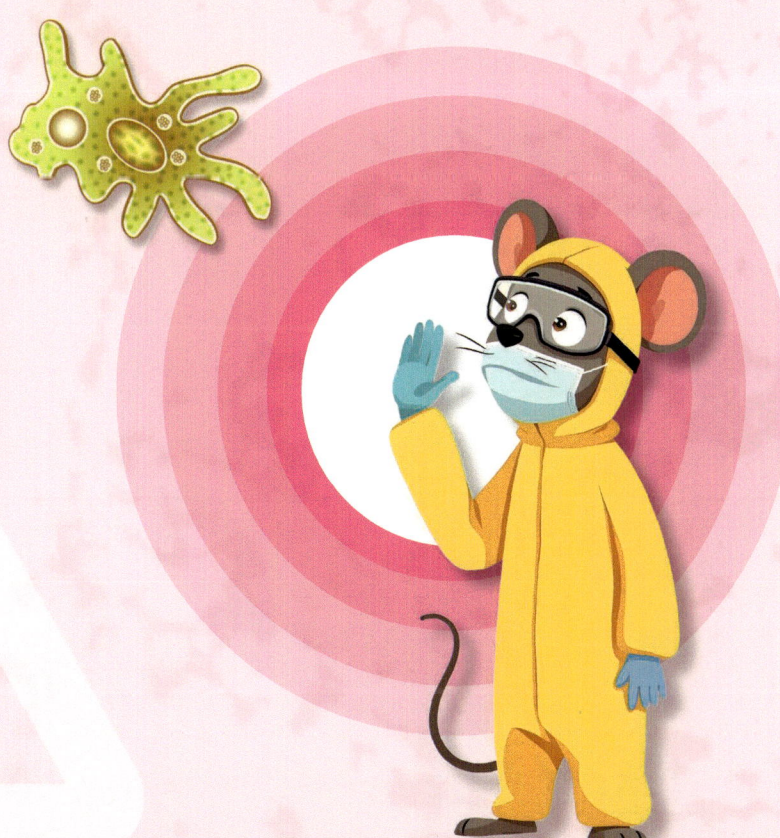

Sneaky Germs

Blood weeping from your eyes? Check. Organs turning to mush? Yep. Ebola is one nasty **virus**. Scientists wanted to know if survivors can still spread it. They tested spit, sweat, and tears. Turns out, Ebola hides for months! Someone who feels fine could still be oozing germs. Yikes!

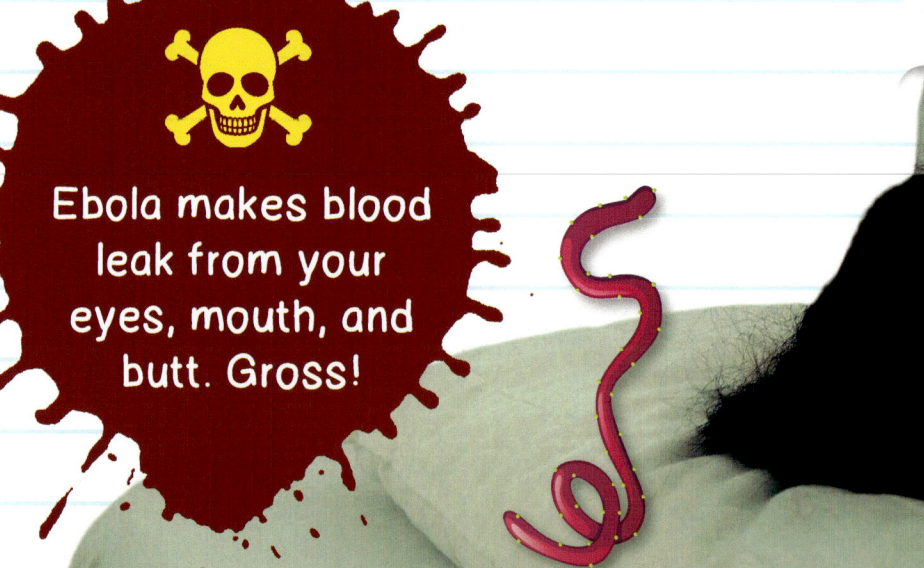

Ebola makes blood leak from your eyes, mouth, and butt. Gross!

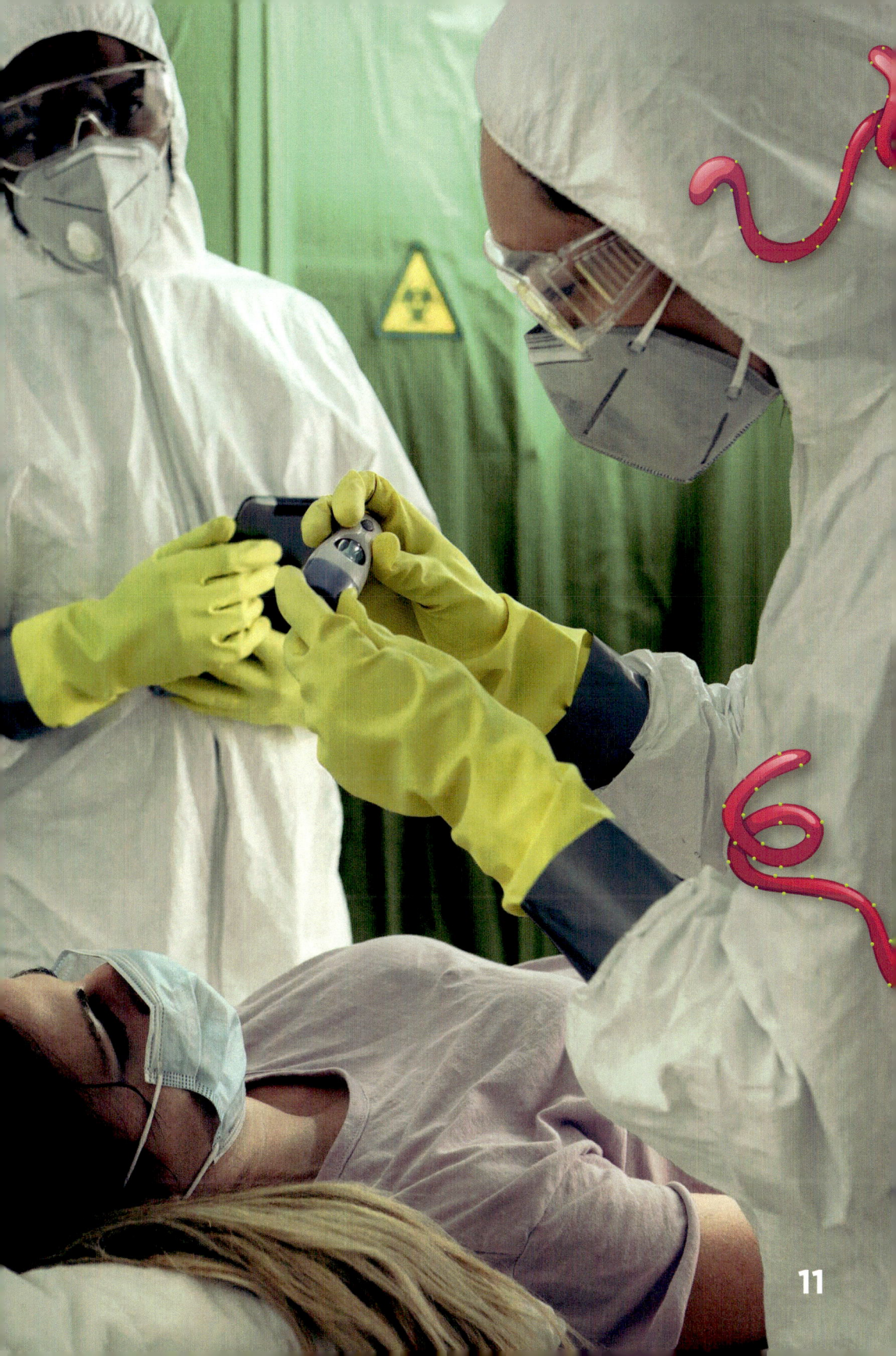

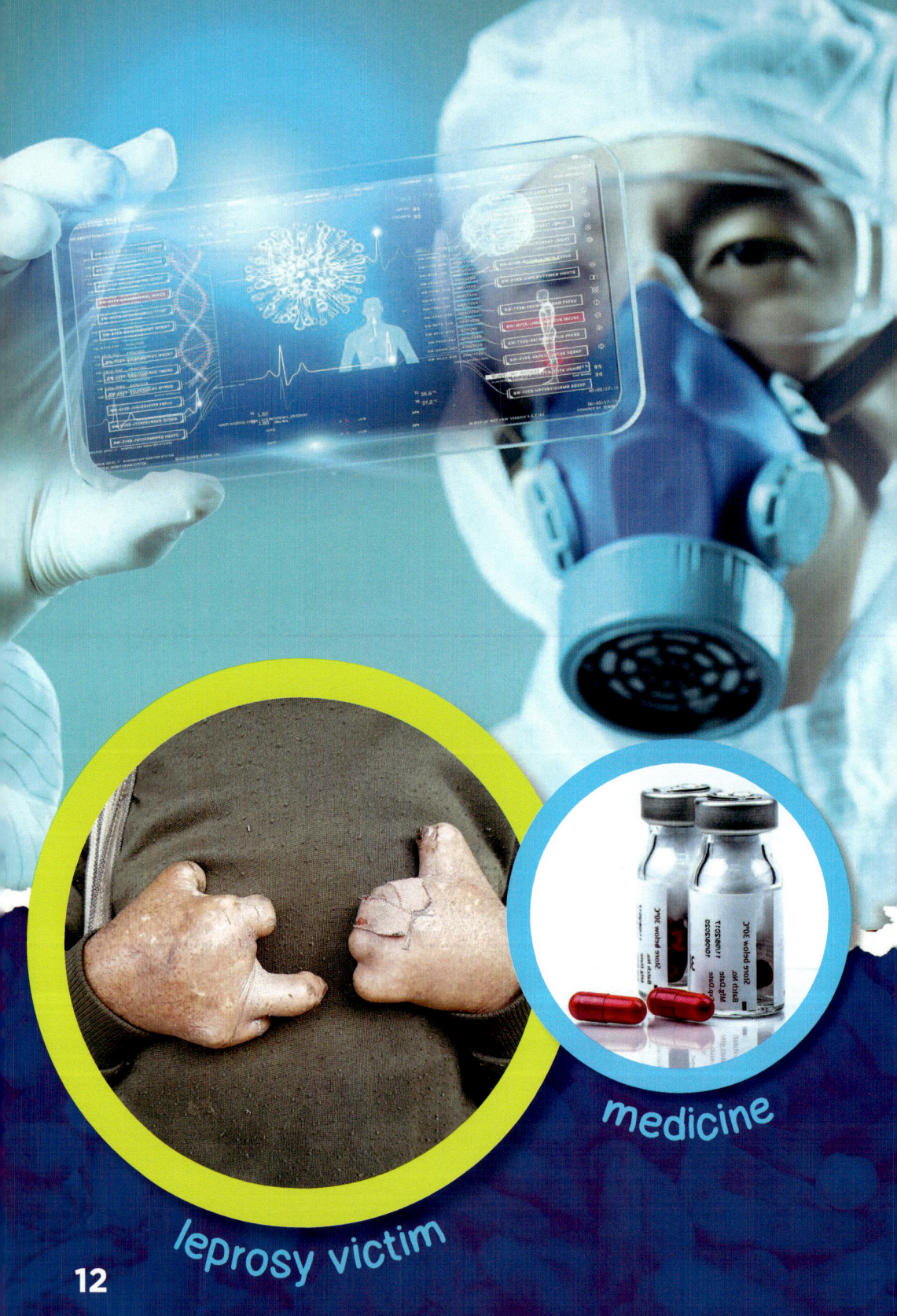

AI to the Rescue!

Leprosy is an infection. It makes your skin look scary. Your fingers and toes go numb. Over time, body parts can rot off. Yuck! Scientists are using **artificial intelligence** (AI). It acts like a disease detective. AI studies germs to find better treatments faster. If it works, leprosy could finally be wiped out. Now that's cool science!

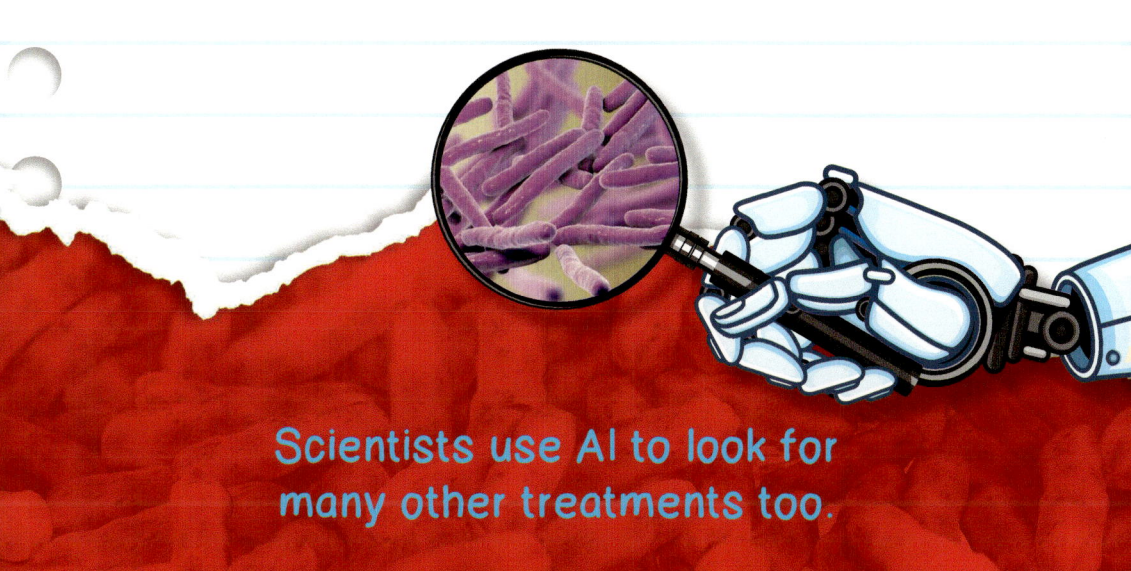

Scientists use AI to look for many other treatments too.

Bye-Bye Bloodsuckers

Mosquitoes spread diseases like malaria and West Nile virus. Scientists are fighting back. They changed mosquito DNA. The female carriers die early. That means fewer babies. Then less disease spreads.

What if human blood was deadly to mosquitoes? It could happen! A drug was given to patients. It usually treats rare diseases. Now it also kills the bugs. They can't digest the blood. They die quickly.

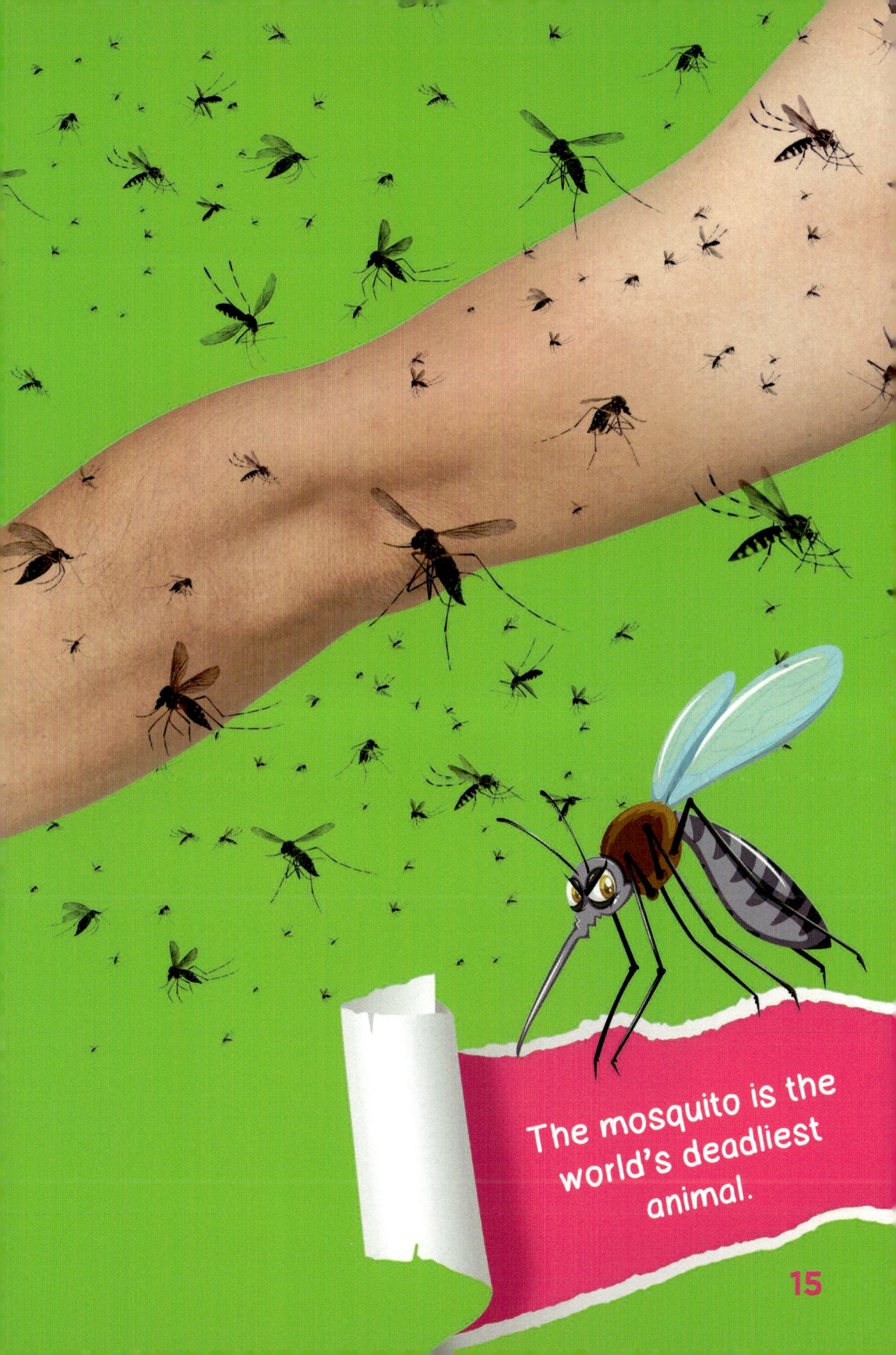

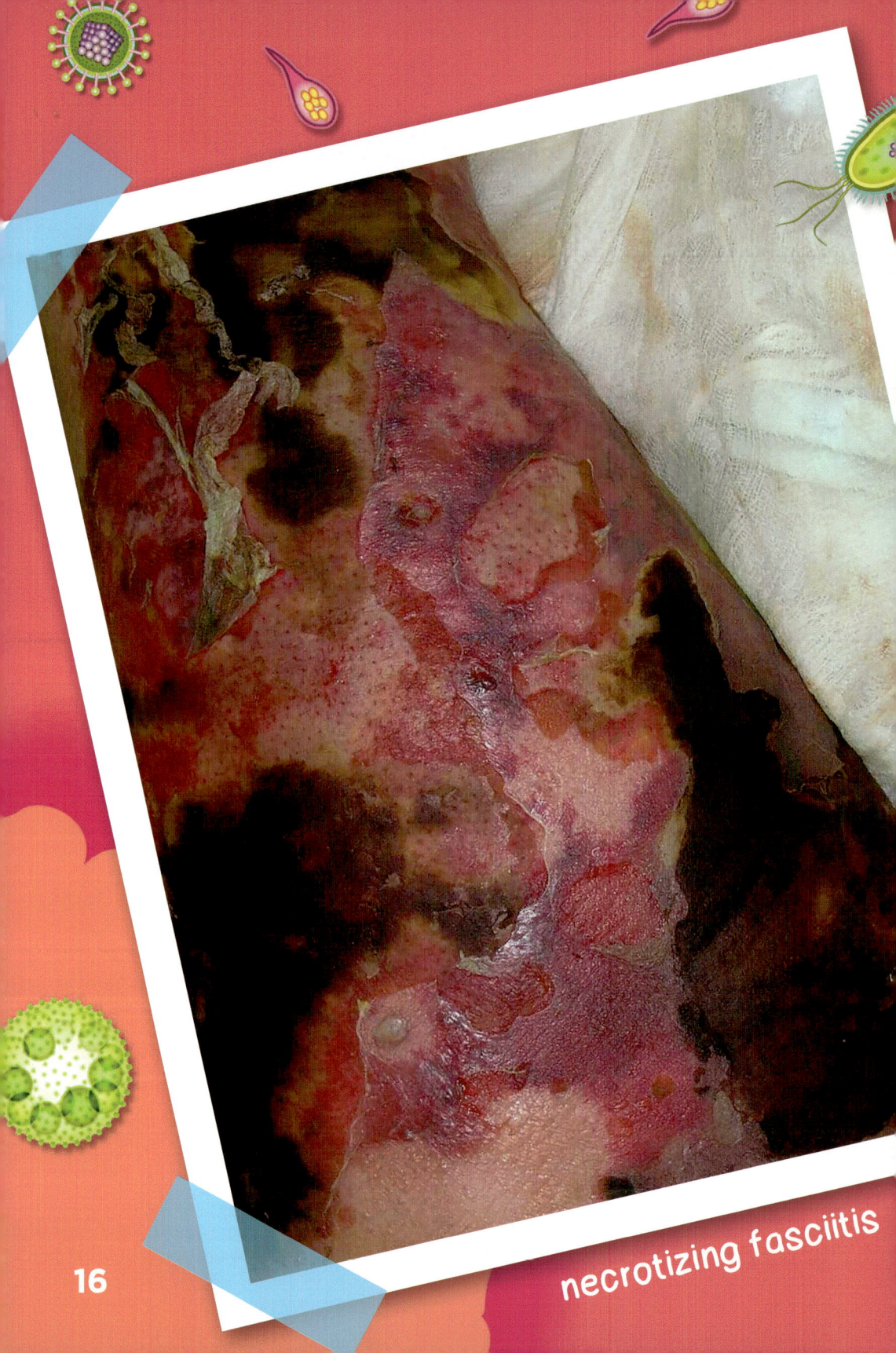
necrotizing fasciitis

Flesh Rot

Flesh-eating **bacteria** can make your skin rot. Then it falls off! Scientists tested a new **antibiotic** on sick mice. Some got the drug. Some didn't. The ones who got it healed fast. The rest? Not so much. This medicine helps stop the infection before the flesh falls off.

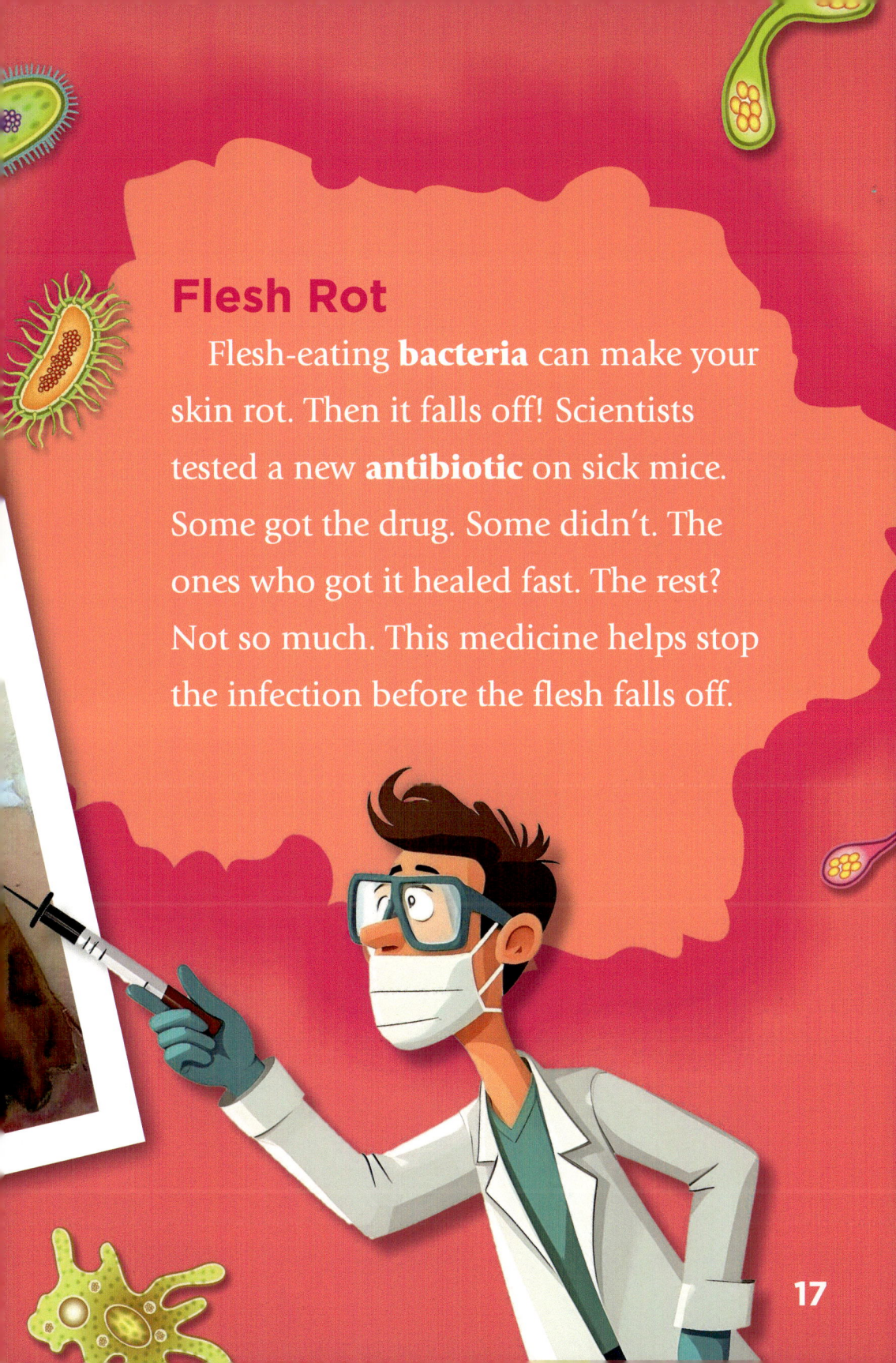

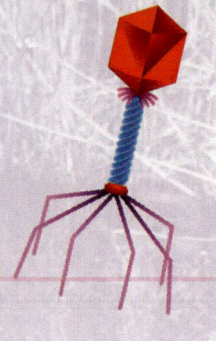

Sewer Viruses

Did you know some treatments come from **sewer** water? It's true! These tiny viruses are called phages. They hunt down and kill bacteria. This could be helpful. Bacteria can become **resistant** to antibiotics. This is a huge threat to people's health. Phages could be a new option. Doctors are still testing how best to use them.

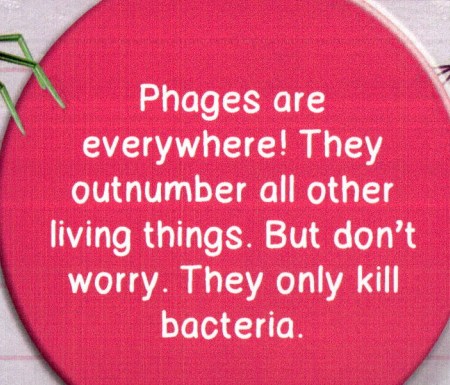

Phages are everywhere! They outnumber all other living things. But don't worry. They only kill bacteria.

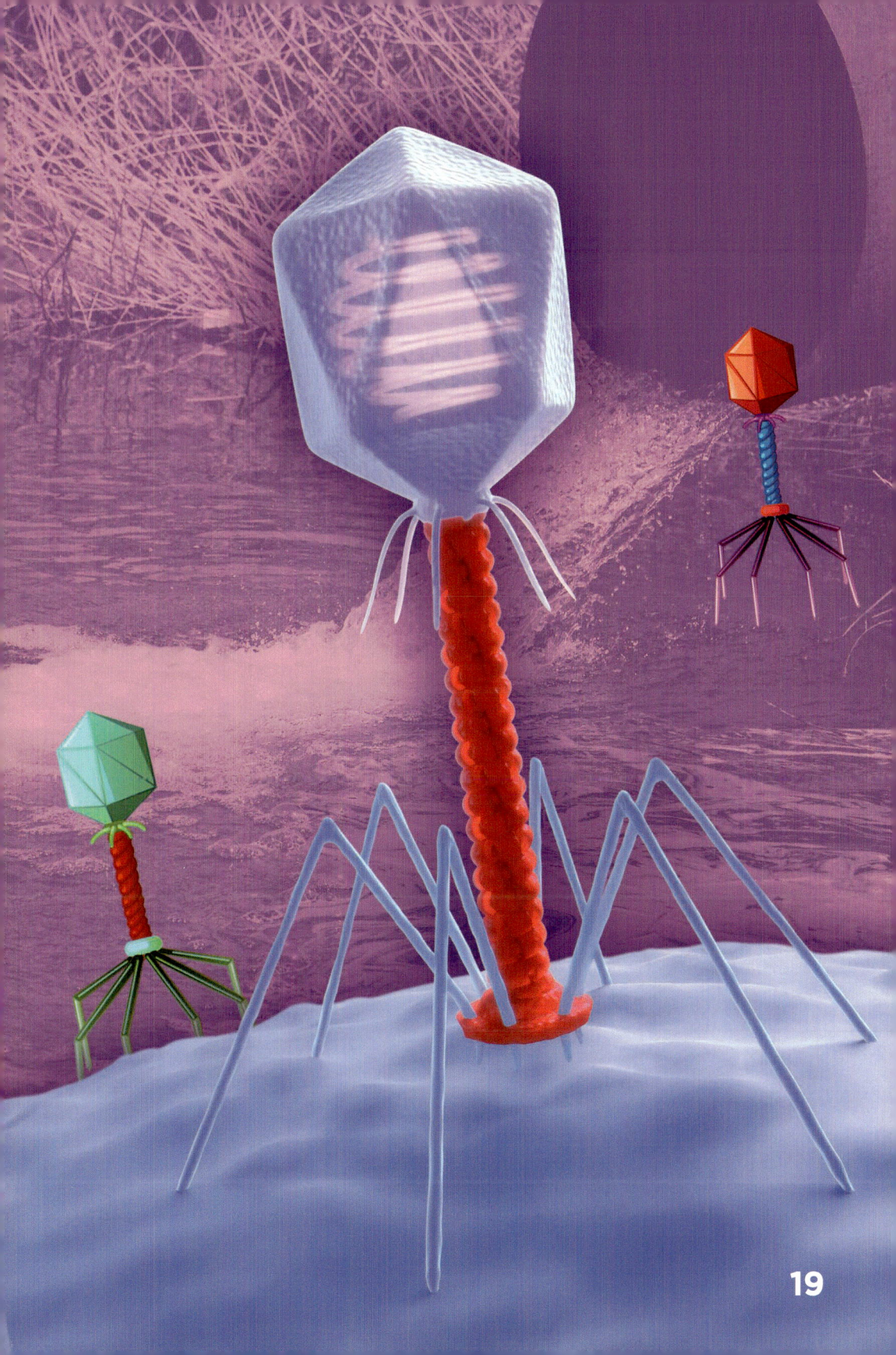

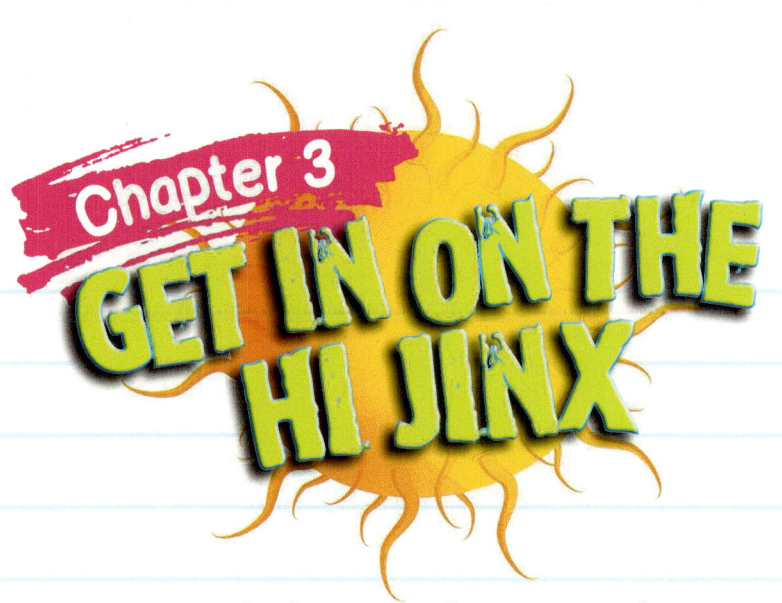

Chapter 3
GET IN ON THE HI JINX

Want to help stop disease and save lives? You could become a laboratory assistant. You'll prepare samples and keep the lab spotless. You'll also help with the experiments. To get this cool gig, you need to study science. Make sure to finish high school. Then you can get on-the-job training to start.

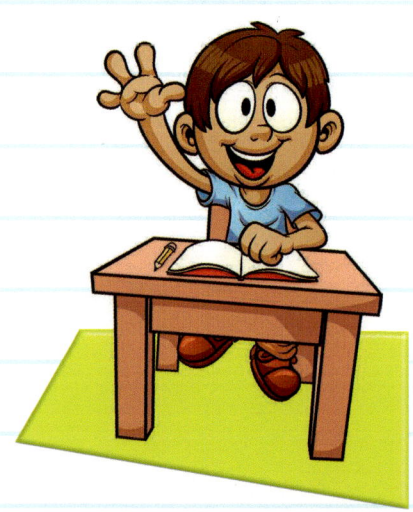

Take It One Step More

1. What can you do to protect yourself from getting sick?

2. Would you want to study diseases? What do you think would be the hardest part?

3. Not all bacteria and viruses are bad. Look up some that are good. How do they help people or animals?

GLOSSARY

antibiotic (an-ti-bahy-OT-ik)—a drug that is used to kill harmful bacteria

artificial intelligence (AHR-tuh-FISH-uhl in-TEL-ih-juhns)—the power of a machine to copy human behavior

bacteria (bak-TEER-ee-uh)—a very small living thing

infect (in-FEKT)—to cause someone or something to become sick or affected with disease

resistant (re-ZIS-tuhnt)—able to withstand the force or effect of something

sewer (SOO-er)—an underground pipe that is used to carry off waste, like poop and pee

symptom (SYMP-tuhm)—a change in the mind or body that means a disease in present

virus (VAHY-ruhs)—a tiny organism that causes a disease

LEARN MORE

BOOKS

Barkman, Rod. *Stop that Germ.* Minneapolis: Bearport Publishing Company, 2025.

Kroe, Kathryn. *What Are Bacteria?* New York: Cavendish Square Publishing, 2023.

WEBSITES

The Deadliest Being on Planet Earth – The Bacteriophage

www.labxchange.org/library/items/lb:LabXchange:a94671ad:video:1

Investigate Diseases and Medicines Science Projects

www.sciencebuddies.org/science-fair-projects/science-projects/investigate-diseases-and-medicines

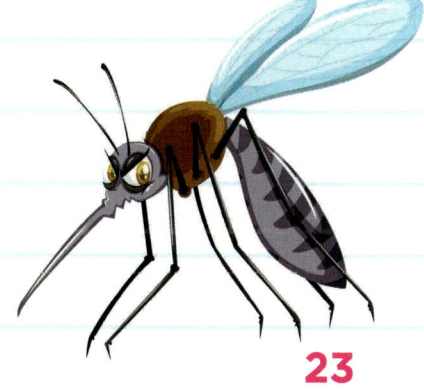

INDEX

A
anthrax, 9

antibiotics, 17, 18

artificial intelligence, 13

B
bacteria, 17, 18

E
ebola, 10

L
laboratory assistants, 20

leprosy, 13

M
mosquitoes, 14, 15

P
phages, 18

S
scabies, 6

V
viruses, 10, 14, 18